T0368176

SEEN KNOWN + HEARD

THE WORKBOOK

Lauren C Shippy

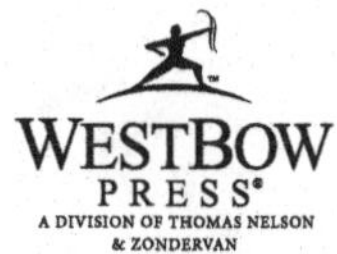

WestBow Press books may be ordered through booksellers or by contacting:

WestBow Press
A Division of Thomas Nelson & Zondervan
1663 Liberty Drive
Bloomington, IN 47403
www.westbowpress.com
844-714-3454

ISBN: 979-8-3850-2959-4 (sc)
ISBN: 979-8-3850-2960-0 (e)

Print information available on the last page.

WestBow Press rev. date: 08/23/2024

THE SLIDESHOW OF THE PEOPLE IN YOUR LIFE

I want you to take a minute and think about the people around you in your life - your family, friends, acquaintances, mailman, barista, assistant, coworker, and anyone else that comes to mind. These people make up a part of your daily life experience. As you think about each one of them in slideshow mode in your mind, what expression is on their face? What phrases do you hear them saying? What is the overall feeling that comes to mind when you think of each person?

As you see this slideshow of photos of all the people that make up your life, I wonder if you have any thoughts that come to mind that surprise you. Things that you have picked up on, maybe an underlying sense that there's more behind the standard greeting. I wonder if right now, you made a list and wrote down the answers to these questions, if you also might hear a phrase for some of them that goes beyond the expression, phrases or feeling. Maybe there's a repeated pattern, concern, or something that you might be hearing them say repeatedly.

This is the start of how practicing seeing, knowing, and hearing others can change everything—and I hope that it does for you too (in a good way). It gave me a new perspective, fresh eyes to see myself and others, that gave me freedom. My hope is that you'll feel the same as you read this, too.

Cheering you on,

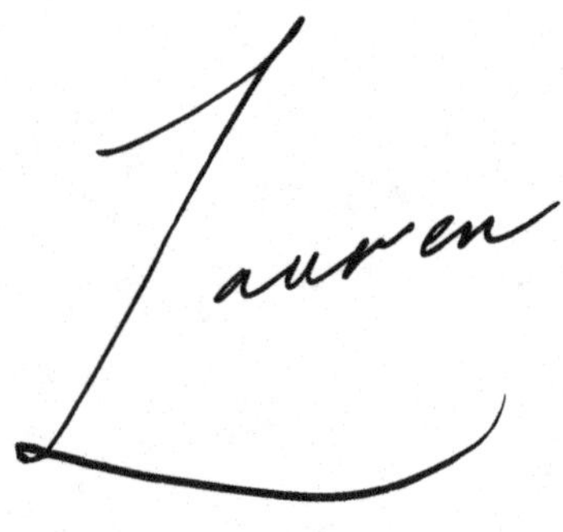

SEEN.
see1 /sē/
verb
to perceive with the eyes; discern visually.

It is said that the eyes are the window to the soul. Can you think of a time when someone's eyes shifted from a soft state to a hard state? Our emotions are often reflected through our eyes. Our "heart condition" shines through our eyes. If we're happy, joyful, generous, well-meaning, or good-spirited, someone can look in our eyes and see it. If we're angry, vengeful, hateful, vindictive, or evil, someone can see that cold, dark look in our eyes and know that something is not right.

Looking into someone else's eyes can tell you a lot about where that person's heart might be at the moment. In fact, science even claims that the eyes produce micro-expressions that give away the intent behind what someone is saying.

If their eyes narrow, they might be skeptical or angry. If their eyes are wide open, they might be scared or alarmed. If their eyes are "smiling," they may feel happy.

Can you picture what you or those around you look like with these expressions? The state of someone's soul can be reflected through their eyes, so if we're looking, we can tell a lot about where someone is before they even say anything at all.

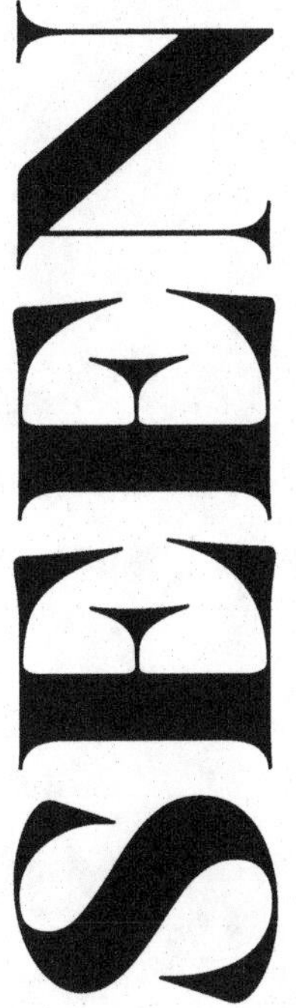

The phrase "the eyes are the window to the soul" has roots in the days of the Roman Empire. As the philosopher Cicero said, "the face is a picture of the mind as the eyes are its interpreter."

Further, some experts, whose jobs require them to study faces, have observed that eyes are the window to the soul because they're the most sincere part of the face.

We don't have any control over our eyes, as opposed to the mouth, for example. When you like something, your pupils dilate involuntarily and give you away, and they contract as a sign of rejection.

As you move through your conversations, start to take notice of the person's eyes as they talk to you. What can you discern as you match their words with their eyes? Do the micro-expressions confirm or deny what they might be saying? If there's a gap, is there a way to ask a question that might unveil more about where they really are?

A THOUGHT

Our body language sends messages that will either strengthen or undermine our ability to be fertilizer. In an effort as fragile as a coalition serving gang-impacted young people, we had to do all we could to build trust among the participants. Did we have real concern for the people around the table? Were we sincerely interested in what others had to say? Were we open to following a collaborative process?

Folded arms, crossed legs, manner of posture—all of these convey something about how we feel about these questions. Equally as important, a self examination of our body language can give us insight into our own motives and heart. At times I have read my own body language and found discomfort, which spurred questions for me to reflect upon: Why am I uncomfortable? What can I do about it? Is it the person, the idea, or some other factor? How am I communicating to others? Is there anything I need to do in response to what my body is telling me?

Keller and Inazu [1]

THE NOTE PAGE

WHERE DO YOU FEEL MOST SEEN?

WHY? WHAT IS IT ABOUT THAT SPACE THAT MAKES YOU FEEL SEEN?

IF THERE ISN'T A PLACE WHERE YOU FEEL SEEN, DO YOU KNOW WHY THAT IS?

IS THERE A WAY YOU'VE BLOCKED CONNECTION OR PREVENTED SAFE PEOPLE FROM REALLY SEEING YOU?

THE NOTE PAGE

HOW CAN YOU FIND THAT FOR YOURSELF: A PLACE, PEOPLE, A CREATOR THAT SEES YOU?

WHO DO YOU THINK FEELS SEEN BY YOU AND WHY?

HOW DO YOU WANT TO PRACTICE SEEING OTHERS AROUND YOU?

REALIZATIONS ON BEING SEEN

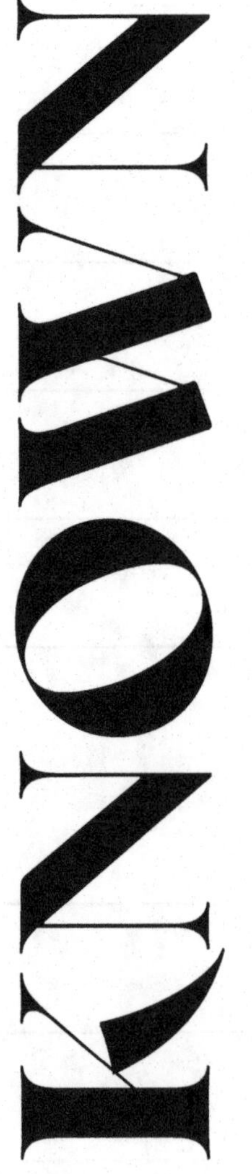

KNOWN.
/nōn/
adjective
recognized, familiar, or within the scope of knowledge.

Known, as we see above, means recognized, familiar, or within the scope of knowledge. When you think about the places or relationships where you're known in your life - do you feel recognized in those spaces?

This is the kind of recognition that acknowledges what you're going through, sees the different parts of your character, and understands some of your deepest desires. It could include the familiar faces that in some way represent comfort to you. The kind of relationships that you are understood, without having to say anything at all.

Maybe it's the people you've grown up with that have known you from the beginning of your life, or your family unit, or friends you have in this stage of life. These places and people might feel like true "home", your safe space, earthly source of refuge and comfort.

As you think about your own life, are there patterns for trying to receive love, such as overachievement, perfectionism, adapting to your audience, or overcompensating? Where do those patterns come from for you? If you experience a lack of feeling known today, is there a "thread", a connection to how you've previously felt not known in the past?

THE NOTE PAGE

WHERE DO YOU FEEL MOST KNOWN?

WHY? WHAT IS IT ABOUT THAT SPACE THAT MAKES YOU FEEL KNOWN?

WHERE ARE YOU UNDERSTOOD WITHOUT USING WORDS?

WHY DO YOU THINK THAT IS?

THE NOTE PAGE

WHAT PLACE AND PEOPLE ARE SAFE SPACES FOR YOU?

IF THERE ISN'T A PLACE WHERE YOU FEEL KNOWN, DO YOU KNOW WHY THAT IS?

IS THERE A WAY YOU'VE BLOCKED CONNECTION OR PREVENTED SAFE PEOPLE FROM REALLY KNOWING YOU?

HOW CAN YOU FIND THAT FOR YOURSELF: A PLACE, PEOPLE, A CREATOR THAT KNOWS YOU?

THE NOTE PAGE

WHO DO YOU THINK FEELS KNOWN BY YOU AND WHY?

HOW DO YOU WANT TO PRACTICE KNOWING OTHERS AROUND YOU?

HOW CAN YOU CREATE A SAFE SPACE FOR OTHERS?

A THOUGHT

Emotional memories are powerful and serve to guide and inform us as we navigate the present and prepare for the future. If you've ever had a drink or taste of something spoiled, you know that emotional memory protects you from doing that again.

Unfortunately, you might unintentionally apply that same principle to relationships, where an implicit or explicit emotional memory cautions you and interferes with your pursuit of having love in your life.

However, sometimes your emotional memories are informing you of a truth that you don't want to acknowledge. The interpretation you make when an emotional memory is activated, in any case, has to be left to your good judgment.

Psychology Today[2]

REALIZATIONS ON BEING KNOWN

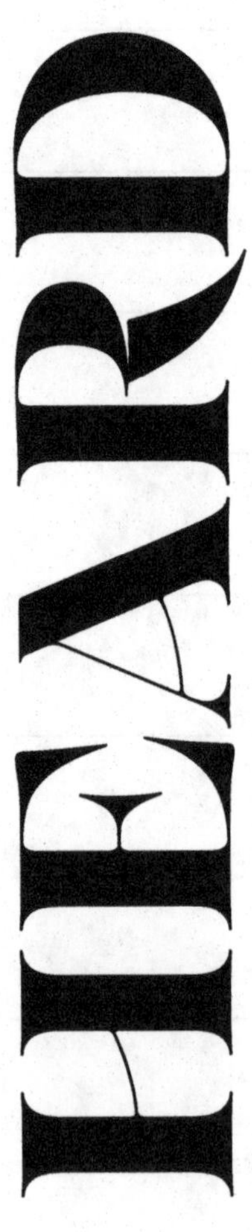

Hearing is translating what is spoken.
HEAR.
/hir/
verb
perceive with the ear the sound made by (someone or something).

I think it's interesting that again we see the word "perceive" within the definition of "hear". A measure of translation has to happen in order for hearing to occur. Our brain has to hear the sound, take it in, translate it, and then trigger a response.

The process of hearing requires translation, much like our sight. The brain translates sounds, so we can produce a response. I'm reminded of being "slow to speak and quick to listen". The pause before responding to check if we've heard the other person correctly is invaluable. A lot of times, our knee jerk response to something can be based on previous patterns, triggers, and assumptions. Our brains naturally live in a state of survival, so our human nature looks to protect ourselves. As we hear something, we must consciously pause to examine our "lens" (how we're viewing the statements we hear through our own filters), so we can form clarifying questions that help us get curious, rather than jump to assumptions.

Instead, let your words come after a pause. Always. Do the same for yourself. There is wisdom in the pause.

Choosing questions over making assumptions always leads to more connection. Choose curiosity over dogmatism. There are very few things that we need to be dogmatic about in this life. Give others the gift of being heard. I promise, it will be a gift to you too.

A THOUGHT

"In times of stress, the best thing we can do for each other is to listen with our ears and our hearts and to be assured that our questions are just as important as our answers."

Fred Rogers [3]

THE NOTE PAGE

DO I HAVE ROOM TO ASK MORE CLARIFYING QUESTIONS IN CONVERSATIONS SO THAT JUDGMENTS OR ASSUMPTIONS DON'T BUILD UP IN RELATIONSHIPS?

DO I PAUSE BEFORE RESPONDING TO CHECK MY RESPONSES?

ARE THERE TIMES WHEN I OR OTHERS HAVE ASKED A "LEADING QUESTION"(ALREADY HAVING THE ANSWER IN MIND, NOT REALLY LISTENING TO THE RESPONSE)?

ARE THERE RELATIONSHIPS WHERE I SEE TRIGGERS OR UNHEALTHY PATTERNS WHERE I CAN'T HEAR OR BE HEARD?

THE NOTE PAGE

WHAT BOUNDARIES NEED TO BE SET IN PLACE?

HOW IS THE TONE OF MY VOICE?

ARE THERE OTHERS THAT COME TO MIND THAT TONE OF VOICE IS GOOD/IRRITATING? WHY?

ARE THERE SITUATIONS THAT COME TO MIND WHERE I CAN IMPROVE MY TONE OF VOICE?

WHAT IS THE TONE OF MY VOICE CONVEYING IN THOSE SITUATIONS (WHAT AM I TRYING TO SAY WITHOUT SAYING AND CAN IT BE RESOLVED/HEALING FOUND)?

REALIZATIONS ON BEING HEARD

"When a person travels through a few years with an organization, or with a partnership, or any other kind of working association, he leaves a "wake" behind in these two areas, task and relationship: What did he accomplish and how did he deal with people? And we can tell a lot about that person from the nature of the wake."

Henry Cloud[4]

Seeing, Knowing + Hearing Yourself.

THE NOTE PAGE

WHAT KIND OF EFFECT DO YOU WANT TO HAVE ON OTHERS AS THEY COME AWAY FROM A CONVERSATION WITH YOU? WHAT DO YOU WANT THEM TO HAVE HEARD?

WHAT WORDS DO YOU SPEAK TO YOURSELF?

WHAT STORY ARE YOU TELLING YOURSELF ABOUT YOURSELF?

ARE THERE ANY WORDS OR PHRASES THAT YOU'VE BEEN SPEAKING TO YOURSELF THAT YOU WANT TO CHANGE?

THE NOTE PAGE

ARE THERE ENVIRONMENTS OR PEOPLE THAT I TEND TO OVERSHARE IN AN EFFORT TO JUSTIFY, DEPEND, OR PROVE YOURSELF?

ARE THERE PLACES WHERE MY IDEOLOGY OR BELIEFS ARE COMING BEFORE CONNECTION WITH OTHERS?

HOW IS MY TONE OF VOICE WITH MYSELF? IF IT'S DEMEANING OR UNKIND, WHY?

WHAT WOULD HAPPEN IF I STARTED BEING KIND TO MYSELF?

A CHALLENGE

**Challenge: For one week, pay extra attention by listening to yourself and the words that you speak to yourself and others. At the end of each day, jot down the things that you would like to change or do differently and why.*

These are some sample questions to get you started:

How was my tone of voice throughout the conversation?

What did I hear myself saying or not saying?

What did I hear the other person saying or not saying?

There is power when we bring subconscious thoughts to the conscious level of thinking because once we start tracking what we're thinking and feeling and how our inputs and conversations are influencing us, we can process and respond to them in a healthy way.

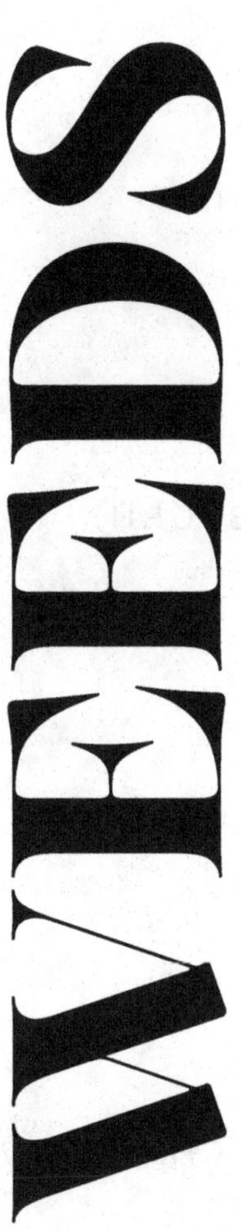

WEED.
/wēd/
noun
a wild plant growing where it is not wanted and in competition with cultivated plants.

Pulling the proverbial weeds in our lives is a refining, healing, freeing process.

Refinement is like peeling an apple, sometimes the skin just doesn't want to budge. We resist hard. We fight tooth and nail not to have something happen or not to have something be the way it is or not to slow down and hear. When it ultimately comes, we realize that surrender was the key all along.

So what do we need to clear out of the way to see, know, and hear others more? The weeds in the way. We'll always be a work in progress, but this is where it gets good. We're going to go places that may be difficult initially, but ultimately can give us newfound freedom, connectedness, and wholeness. That's our goal. In order to get to this place, we've got to clear out the weeds in the way.

What has infiltrated your heart that's causing anguish, anxiety, bitterness, grief, sorrow, distress, depression, sadness, anger, or hopelessness? Is it parked there and how long has it camped out there? What are the impacts of holding it on your health (mental, physical, emotional, spiritual)? Has holding these emotions benefitted you in any way?

Let's look at some specific weeds in the way and how they can impact us. As you read through these, think about your own life experiences and what weeds you might want to pull from your life.

WEED #1: STUBBORNESS

STUBBORNNESS IS CLINGING TO SOMETHING THAT HAS LONG PASSED.

IT'S THE UNYIELDING REFUSAL TO CHANGE YOUR MIND ABOUT A SITUATION OR PERSON THAT NEGATIVELY AFFECTED YOU. IT'S EASY TO BE STUBBORN ABOUT MANY THINGS, BUT THE LONGER I LIVE AND EXPERIENCE HURT IN THIS WORLD, I'M FINDING THAT THERE ARE VERY FEW THINGS THAT ARE ACTUALLY WORTH BEING STUBBORN ABOUT.

I WOULD CALL THIS A FORM OF LEGALISM THAT KEEPS US GLUED TO THE LETTER OF THE LAW INSTEAD OF ITS SPIRIT. YOU MAY FALL PREY TO THIS IF YOU FIND YOURSELF SAYING THE FOLLOWING THINGS ABOUT YOUR BELIEFS:

"I DO IT THIS WAY BECAUSE I'VE ALWAYS DONE IT THIS WAY."
"I'M SUCCESSFUL BECAUSE I ALWAYS TIE MY SHOES THIS WAY."
"YOU HAVE TO GO TO THE GROCERY STORE USING THIS ROAD."
"ON TUESDAYS, WE MUST HAVE TACOS."

QUESTIONS FOR REFLECTION

WHAT COMES TO MIND FOR YOU WHEN YOU READ THIS?

ARE THERE AREAS OF YOUR LIFE WHERE YOU FEEL STUBBORN?
IS IT HELPING OR HINDERING YOU?

IF IT'S HELPING YOU, HOW?

IF IT'S HINDERING YOU, WHY? WHAT WOULD YOU LIKE TO CHANGE?

WEED #2: CONTROL

CONTROL CAN GIVE US A FALSE SENSE OF SECURITY. CONTROLLING OUR SCHEDULES, TIME, AND EVEN OTHER PEOPLE IS SOMETHING WE ATTEMPT TO DO IN SOME WAY EVERY DAY. CONTROL CAN MAKE US FEEL LIKE WE'RE ON TOP OF THINGS—LIKE WE'VE GOT IT TOGETHER. WE PULL THINGS IN A LITTLE TIGHTER (MOSTLY SUBCONSCIOUSLY) BECAUSE WE THINK DOING SO WILL GIVE US A SENSE OF PEACE OR SECURITY. THE PROBLEM WITH CONTROL, THOUGH, IS THAT IT'S AN ILLUSION MOST OF THE TIME. WE DON'T ACTUALLY HAVE CONTROL OVER MUCH AT ALL, OTHER THAN OURSELVES AND OUR OWN REACTIONS.

QUESTIONS FOR REFLECTION

WHAT AREAS OF CONTROL DO YOU TEND TO CLING TO?

WHAT MIGHT YOU THINK ABOUT RELEASING?

IF YOU WERE TO RELEASE IT, HOW WOULD THAT FEEL FOR YOU? WHY?

WHAT'S STOPPING YOU FROM RELEASING CONTROL?

WEED #3: UNFORGIVENESS

"FORGIVENESS HAS NOTHING TO DO WITH ABSOLVING A CRIMINAL OF HIS CRIME. IT HAS EVERYTHING TO DO WITH RELIEVING ONESELF OF THE BURDEN OF BEING A VICTIM—LETTING GO OF THE PAIN AND TRANSFORMING ONESELF FROM VICTIM TO SURVIVOR."
C.R. STRAHAN[5]

THE ONLY PERSON THAT UNFORGIVENESS HOLDS CAPTIVE IS YOU. IN PREPARATION FOR PRACTICING A LIFESTYLE OF SEEING, KNOWING, AND HEARING OTHERS, A REGULAR RHYTHM OF RELEASING OTHERS AND FORGIVING THEM WILL SET US FREE. FORGIVENESS IS SIMPLY AN ACKNOWLEDGEMENT THAT YOU NO LONGER HOLD THE OFFENSE AGAINST THEM; YOU RELEASE THEM TO GOD TO DEAL WITH THEM IN HIS TIME AND IN HIS WAY. IN OTHER WORDS, WE NO LONGER CARRY THE BURDEN OF SETTING THE RECORD STRAIGHT, RIGHTING THEIR WRONG, OR HOLDING THEM TO EXPECTATIONS OF REPENTANCE OR JUSTICE. WE SET THEM FREE TO LET THE OFFENDER WORK THEIR OWN STUFF OUT.

QUESTIONS FOR REFLECTION

WHERE DO YOU FEEL "HELD CAPTIVE" BY FORGIVENESS?

WHAT IS IT COSTING ME TO FORGIVE THEM?

WHAT WILL I GAIN BY FORGIVING THEM?

WHAT WOULD IT LOOK LIKE FOR ME TO PRACTICE FORGIVENESS REGULARLY?

WEED #4: BITTERNESS

BITTERNESS, OR RESENTMENT, IS ANGER COMPOUNDED OVER TIME. BITTER ROOTS RUN DEEP. BITTERNESS DOESN'T JUST HAPPEN ON THE FIRST OFFENSE, IT SIMMERS SLOWLY AND WITH EACH OFFENSE, IT GROWS. MY THERAPIST USED TO SAY THAT BITTERNESS IS LIKE A CUT. THE FIRST TIME YOU GET A CUT, IT CAN HEAL PRETTY QUICKLY. THE SECOND, THIRD, AND FOURTH TIME YOU HIT IT IN THAT SAME PLACE, IT'S GOING TO TAKE LONGER TO HEAL BECAUSE THE WOUND NOW RUNS DEEPER. BITTERNESS IS THE SAME; EACH TIME SOMEONE HURTS US USING THE SAME PATTERN, IN A SIMILAR SCENARIO, OR LEAVES US WITH THE SAME FEELING, IT DRIVES THAT BITTERNESS OR RESENTMENT DOWN DEEPER.

QUESTIONS FOR REFLECTION

WHAT BITTERNESS HAS BEEN "SIMMERING" SLOWLY IN MY LIFE?

WHEN DID IT START (WHAT'S THE ROOT)?

WHAT IS IT COSTING ME TO HANG ON TO BITTERNESS?

WHAT WILL I GAIN BY RELEASING IT?

WHERE DO I/CAN I FIND A SAFE SPACE IF I WANT TO RELEASE SOME OF MY BITTERNESS?

WEED #5: ANGER

ASIDE FROM SOCIAL MEDIA, MANY OF US HAVE EXPERIENCED TURMOIL IN OUR CLOSE RELATIONSHIPS OVER THE LAST SEVERAL YEARS. NOT TO MENTION ALL OF THE ANGER MANY OF US HAVE EXPERIENCED IN OUR LIFETIME, DUE TO LIFE SITUATIONS, MISSED EXPECTATIONS, AND FEELING DISRESPECTED OR MISTREATED OR UNNOTICED BY OTHERS. SO IMAGINE THESE THREE "LAYERS" OF ANGER EACH OF US IS CARRYING AROUND: SOCIAL MEDIA NOISE, THE CURRENT CLIMATE IN OUR WORLD, OUR PERSONAL EXPERIENCES, AND RELATIONSHIP TENSION. IT CAN FEEL AS YOU READ THIS THAT ALL HOPE IS LOST, BUT IT'S NOT. RECOGNIZING IT IS THE FIRST STEP. YOU'LL NOW START TO RECOGNIZE THESE LAYERS SHOWING UP IN YOUR LIFE. BUT WHAT DO YOU DO WITH IT?

QUESTIONS FOR REFLECTION

WHAT HAS MADE ME ANGRY IN THE PAST?

WHAT IS MAKING ME ANGRY RIGHT NOW?

HOW IS THAT ANGER AFFECTING ME?

WEED #5: ANGER

WHAT IS THE ANGER TELLING ME (ANGER IS A SIGNAL THAT SOMETHING NEEDS CHANGE)?

WHAT TOOLS CAN I USE TO HELP ME VENT (TALKING TO A TRUSTED FRIEND, PUNCHING BAG, A RUN, ETC.)

HOW CAN I MAKE TIME TO NOTICE MY ANGER AND VENT ON A REGULAR BASIS?

WEED #6: ASSUMPTIONS + JUDGEMENTS

HAVE YOU EVER BEEN TALKING TO SOMEONE AND YOU'RE NOT FULLY HEARING WHAT THEY'RE SAYING IN THE MOMENT BECAUSE YOU HEARD THEM SAY A PARTICULAR WORD OR PHRASE AND YOUR MIND STARTED TO AUTOMATICALLY "CLASSIFY" WHAT THEY'VE SAID INTO A CATEGORY? ASSUMPTIONS CAN HAPPEN QUICKLY, SO THEY'RE TRICKY TO KEEP TRACK OF UNLESS WE REALLY ASSESS OUR THOUGHTS REGULARLY: WE CAN MAKE THEM IN A SPLIT SECOND, WITHOUT EVEN KNOWING IT.

ASSUMPTIONS ARE OFTEN UNPROMPTED AND BASED ON A NUMBER OF DIVERSE THINGS SUCH AS OUR PAST EXPERIENCES IN LIFE, PEOPLE WE KNOW LIKE THEM, OUR POLITICAL OR RELIGIOUS BELIEFS, OUR NEWS AND SOCIAL MEDIA FEEDS, AND SO MUCH MORE. AS WE'RE SEEING PEOPLE THROUGHOUT THE DAY, WHETHER WORDS ARE USED OR NOT, WE'RE PROBABLY MAKING A WHOLE BUNCH OF ASSUMPTIONS ABOUT THOSE PEOPLE—EVERYTHING FROM SURFACE LEVEL DEMOGRAPHICS LIKE THEIR SOCIOECONOMIC STATUS, SEXUAL ORIENTATION, BACKGROUND AND UPBRINGING, AND THEIR EDUCATION LEVEL. WE ALSO MIGHT BE SUBCONSCIOUSLY OR CONSCIOUSLY MAKING ASSUMPTIONS ABOUT THEIR PHILOSOPHIES AND WORLDVIEW SUCH AS THEIR FAITH, POLITICAL ORIENTATION, OR THEIR STANCE ON SOCIAL ISSUES. WE ALL HAVE BIASES—WHETHER WE ACKNOWLEDGE THEM CONSCIOUSLY OR NOT. WE ALL HAVE TRIGGERS THAT CREATE ASSOCIATIONS WITH PAST WOUNDS AND HURTS.

QUESTIONS FOR REFLECTION

WHO IS COMING TO MIND FOR ME AS I THINK ABOUT ASSUMPTIONS AND JUDGEMENTS?

WHAT RELATIONSHIP(S) HAVE I STRUGGLED WITH MAKING ASSUMPTIONS AND JUDGEMENTS?

WHAT ASSUMPTIONS AND JUDGEMENTS HAVE I MADE ABOUT MYSELF?

WEED #6: ASSUMPTIONS + JUDGEMENTS

WHAT SITUATIONS LEAD ME TO TEND TO THINK TOO QUICKLY OR SPEAK BEFORE I THINK?

AM I SEEKING TO CONTROL SOMEONE ELSE OR MYSELF BY MAKING ASSUMPTIONS OR JUDGEMENTS THAT CAN MAKE ME FEEL A FALSE SENSE OF "SAFETY"?

WHAT MIGHT I BE MISSING BY ASSUMING WITHOUT VERIFYING THOUGHTS ABOUT MYSELF AND OTHERS?

WHAT WOULD IT LOOK LIKE IF I RELEASED THOSE ASSUMPTIONS AND JUDGEMENTS? WHAT WOULD IT GIVE ME?

WHAT WOULD HELP ME BE MORE AWARE OF MY FORMATION OF ASSUMPTIONS AND JUDGEMENTS TOWARD MYSELF AND OTHERS MOVING FORWARD?

WEED #7: LACK OF SELF AWARENESS

SELF-AWARENESS MAY SEEM COUNTERINTUITIVE TO SEEING, HEARING, AND KNOWING OTHERS, BUT I BELIEVE THAT WORKING ON OURSELVES IS ACTUALLY FOUNDATIONAL TO BEING ABLE TO CONNECT WELL WITH OTHERS. WE ALL WANT TO BE SEEN OURSELVES; ONCE WE FIGURE OUT THE MOMENTS THROUGHOUT OUR LIVES WHERE WE'VE WANTED TO BE SEEN OR KNOWN OR HEARD AND HAVEN'T BEEN, WE CAN START TO BECOME AWARE OF THE THINGS THAT NOW TRIGGER US. MAYBE IT'S THE RELATIONSHIPS THAT BOTHER US, THE SPECIFIC WORDS, PHRASES, OR HABITS OF OUR SIGNIFICANT OTHERS THAT DON'T SIT WELL WITH US, THE COWORKER WHO NEVER LOOKS AT US WHEN HE TALKS, AND I'M SURE YOU CAN THINK OF A FEW MORE PERSONAL EXAMPLES. ONCE WE WORK THROUGH THESE TRIGGERS, WE WILL GAIN UNDERSTANDING AND A LARGER PERSPECTIVE OF WHY THESE THINGS HAVE BOTHERED US SO MUCH. ONCE WE HAVE AN UNDERSTANDING OF THOSE TRIGGERS, THEY WON'T BECOME KRYPTONITE FOR US ANYMORE; WE CAN DISASSOCIATE FROM THEM IN A HEALTHY WAY IN ORDER TO TRY TO SEE, HEAR, AND KNOW OTHER PEOPLE.

QUESTIONS FOR REFLECTION

WHERE HAVE I NOT BEEN HONEST WITH MYSELF?

WHY IS IT HARD?

WHAT EMOTIONS DOES IT BRING UP FOR ME?

WHAT ARE THESE EMOTIONS TELLING ME?

WEED #7: LACK OF SELF AWARENESS

WHAT HAVE BEEN MY EXAMPLES OF SELF AWARENESS GROWING UP/THROUGHOUT MY LIFE?

HAVE I SEEN THIS MODELED?

HOW CAN I BE PRESENT WITH MYSELF ON A DAILY BASIS?

WHAT HAS "HELD ME CAPTIVE"—SOMETHING I HAVEN'T SEEN BEFORE THIS MOMENT?

WHAT CAN I DO ABOUT WHAT I'VE DISCOVERED HERE?

WEED #8: PRIDE

PRIDE ALWAYS PREVENTS US FROM SEEING, KNOWING, AND HEARING OUR TRUE SELVES (AND OTHERS) BECAUSE SOMETIMES WE DON'T LIKE WHAT'S BEHIND THE CURTAIN SO WE FEEL THE NEED TO PUT ON A SHOW. INEVITABLY, THIS FUELS OUR DESIRE TO PUT ON A MASK SO PEOPLE CAN'T SEE US AS WE REALLY ARE, BUT IN THE PROCESS OF DOING SO WE LOSE THE OPPORTUNITY TO SEE, HEAR, AND KNOW OTHERS. IT PREVENTS US FROM BEING APPROACHABLE AND RELATABLE TO OTHERS. I WONDER IF THE STRUGGLE WITH PRIDE COMES FROM A NEED THAT ALL OF US HAVE FOR SIGNIFICANCE.

PERHAPS PRIDE STEMS FROM A LACK OF BEING SEEN, KNOWN, AND HEARD EARLIER IN OUR LIVES. AS A RESULT, A HOLE CREATES AN EMPTY SPACE LONGING FOR THE ACKNOWLEDGEMENT WE SO BADLY WANTED. WE FELT LIKE WE WERE DESPERATELY TRYING TO BE HEARD, TO BE RECOGNIZED AS AN INDIVIDUAL HUMAN, AND TO BE KNOWN. AS IS THE CASE WITH MANY OF OUR "WEEDS IN THE WAY, " RECOGNITION OF THE DEEP ROOT CAUSE STARTS THE PROCESS OF UNCOVERING WHY AND WHERE PRIDE CREEPS IN. WHEN WE KNOW THIS, WE CAN START TO TAKE NOTICE OF THE PLACES, SITUATIONS, AND RELATIONSHIPS WHERE OUR NEED TO PROVE KEEPS SHOWING UP. WE CAN GIVE OURSELVES THE GIFT OF STEPPING OUT OF THOSE SPACES WHEN WE NEED TO.

QUESTIONS FOR REFLECTION

WHERE DO I SEE PRIDE SHOWING UP IN MY LIFE?

IS PRIDE JUST A COVER FOR BLOCKING ME FROM LETTING PEOPLE INTO MY WORLD?

AM I AFRAID TO LET THEM IN FOR FEAR THAT THEY MAY NOT LIKE WHO I REALLY AM?

WEED #8: PRIDE

WHY WOULDN'T THEY REALLY LIKE WHO I AM? WHAT PART OF ME?

IS THERE A SPACE IN ME THAT IS LONGING FOR ACKNOWLEDGEMENT? WHERE?

IS PRIDE BLOCKING ME FROM SEEING, HEARING, AND KNOWING OTHERS? RECALL A SPECIFIC TIME THAT THIS HAPPENED AND WRITE ABOUT IT.

HOW DO I WANT TO MOVE FORWARD IN LIGHT OF WHAT I'VE DISCOVERED HERE?

WEED #9: SKEPTICISM

SKEPTICISM HOLDS A POSTURE OF DOUBT, UNCERTAINTY, AND CRITICISM. IT CAN STEAL OUR SENSE OF WONDER. I PICTURE A BALLOON'S AIR SLOWLY BEING LET OUT UNTIL THERE'S NOTHING LEFT. SKEPTICISM DOES THAT TO OUR SOULS. IT QUITE LITERALLY SUCKS THE LIFE OUT OF US, IF WE LET IT.

MAYBE YOU'RE READING THIS AND YOU'RE THINKING, THERE'S GOOD REASON I FEEL SKEPTICAL ABOUT THE POSSIBILITY OF BEING SEEN, KNOWN, AND HEARD. I COMPLETELY UNDERSTAND THAT. YOU'VE BEEN THROUGH HARD THINGS, YOU'VE EXPERIENCED TRAUMA, PEOPLE IN YOUR LIFE HAVE COMPLETELY CRUSHED YOU WITH BETRAYAL AND LIES, WHILE OTHERS HAVE ROBBED YOU OF JOY AND MIGHT AS WELL HAVE RIPPED YOUR HEART OUT. I GET IT AND I SEE YOU, BUT LET ME TELL YOU SOMETHING. YOU DON'T HAVE TO LET THOSE PEOPLE WIN. BY MAINTAINING A POSTURE OF SKEPTICISM, YOU ARE LETTING YOUR ENEMY WIN.

QUESTIONS FOR REFLECTION

WHERE DO I FIND MY SKEPTICISM REARING ITS HEAD? (WHAT PEOPLE, SITUATIONS, REPEATED PATTERNS, HUMOR)

WHAT IS UNDERNEATH THAT SKEPTICISM?

WHAT IS IT THAT I REALLY WANT TO SAY?

WEED #9: SKEPTICISM

WHEN WAS MY SENSE OF WONDER STOLEN FROM ME THROUGHOUT MY LIFE?

HOW HAS MY SKEPTICISM HELD ME BACK IN MY LIFE?

HOW CAN I START TO RECLAIM SOME HOPE IN MY LIFE?

WEED #10: ______________________________

THIS SPACE IS LEFT BLANK FOR YOU; CHANCES ARE, AS YOU STARTED UPROOTING SOME OF THESE WEEDS, YOU MAY HAVE FOUND SOME OTHERS TRYING TO HANG AROUND. YOU'RE ALREADY HERE, SO YOU MIGHT AS WELL KICK AS MANY OUT AS POSSIBLE.

QUESTIONS FOR REFLECTION

LIST OUT ANY OTHER "WEEDS IN THE WAY" FOR YOU:

WHAT PAIN OR HARDSHIP HAS HOLDING ONTO THESE WEEDS CAUSED YOU?

WHAT ARE YOU COMMITTED TO RELEASING TODAY?

WEEDS IN THE WAY RECAP

WE NEED TO UPROOT WEEDS IN ORDER TO TRULY SEE OURSELVES AND OTHERS AS WE ARE, IF WE DON'T, IT KEEPS US TRAPPED AND LESS CONNECTED. I DON'T KNOW ABOUT YOU, BUT I GET PRETTY MAD ABOUT THE THOUGHT THAT FALSE BELIEFS, NEGATIVE TRACKS, AND PAST EXPERIENCES CAN TELL US A STORY INSIDE OF OUR MINDS THAT'S NOT ACCURATE. WE'RE HELD CAPTIVE TO THE SURFACE LEVEL OF WHO WE THINK WE ARE; A LOT OF TIMES, THOSE PERCEPTIONS ARE NOT CORRECT. THOSE LIES CAN HOLD US BACK FROM OPERATING IN OUR PURPOSE ALONG THE WAY. THEY CAN HOLD US BACK FROM ENGAGING IN NEW RELATIONSHIPS OR OPPORTUNITIES AND EXPERIENCING JOY.

IF WE DON'T KNOW OURSELVES, WE CAN'T KNOW OTHERS. IF WE LACK SELF-AWARENESS, WE WILL LACK AWARENESS OF WHAT OTHERS ARE WANTING OR NEEDING, MAKING IT DIFFICULT FOR US TO HAVE CONNECTION THAT BRINGS FULFILLMENT. CONNECTION DRIVES US AS HUMANS.

WHEN WE CLEAR OUT THE WEEDS IN THE WAY, WE GIVE OURSELVES THE GIFT OF FREEDOM. WHEN WE'RE FREE, WE CAN SEE AND HEAR CLEARLY; IT OPENS UP NEW PERSPECTIVES, UNLOCKS EMPATHY, AND ULTIMATELY HEALS OUR HEARTS.

QUESTIONS FOR REFLECTION

WHICH OF THE WEEDS THAT WE DISCUSSED FEELS THE MOST PERSONAL TO YOU?

TAKE A MOMENT AND LIST THEM OUT, ALONG WITH SOME POTENTIAL BLINDSPOTS.

WEEDS IN THE WAY RECAP

NEXT, LIST OUT SOME SITUATIONS THAT “TIPPED YOU OFF” TO THESE POTENTIAL BLINDSPOTS.

IS THERE A FRIEND, COUNSELOR, OR MENTOR THAT YOU CAN SHARE THESE WITH AND ASK FOR FEEDBACK? WRITE THEIR NAME DOWN AND ASK THEM IF THEY’RE OPEN TO HAVING A BLINDSPOT CONVERSATION.

The Framework

MAKE SPACE
LISTEN
UNDERSTAND
COMMUNICATE

When I wrote the outline for the Seen, Known, and Heard framework, the four steps I'm about to share with you sounded too simple. As I looked closer, I realized that, as per usual, there's a lot more beneath the surface. As we examined the weeds in the way, there were words like stubbornness and unforgiveness that you have known for years, but you may have seen them differently as you read them in this book. Much like a kaleidoscope, as you turn the wheel on the end of it, the frame changes. As we move throughout our lives, depending on what we've been through and where we are, things hit differently.

As you read through this framework, picture yourself sitting next to an old radio in a fancy chair (like they used to before TV), trying to tune into whatever the nightly program might be. It's crackling and you have to get that dial just right to hear clearly and tune it to the one available station. My hope is that as you read this, you can picture yourself tuning that radio into your station to hear yourself clearly. Then, in turn, that you can tune into the station of others when you need to.

MAKE SPACE

SPACE.
/spās/
noun
a continuous area or expanse which is free, available, or unoccupied.

If you think about your average day and envision a pie chart of your time, what things would be on it and what percentage of your day do they consume? These might include cooking, cleaning, taking care of kids or family, working out, working, texting, social media browsing, talking on the phone, running errands, reading, listening to podcasts, etc.

Now, figure out how many of the activities on that pie chart stem from wanting a distraction. I said stems from because I think it's important to investigate the reason for seeking out distractions. Sometimes, we don't even realize that we are distracting ourselves. This often comes in the form of procrastination, avoidance, fear, or others encouraging us to remain in a state of distraction because it benefits them.

There are lots of things you can do to take back your time, and only you can determine what you need. Just give yourself the gift of time. Time makes space for you to feel human again, for you to check in and assess how you're really doing, and to give yourself the break you need.

MAKE SPACE

WHAT DO I FEEL CONSUMES TOO MUCH OF MY DAY?

WHAT CONSUMES TOO LITTLE?

WHAT AM I FEELING GUILT OR SHAME ABOUT RIGHT NOW, IN REGARDS TO MY TIME?

IS IT VALID?

IF IT IS, WHAT CHANGES DO I WANT TO MAKE IN LIGHT OF THESE DISCOVERIES?

IF IT ISN'T, WHAT "WEED" DO I NEED TO UPROOT TO CLEAR OUT THAT SHAME OR FALSE GUILT?

MAKE SPACE

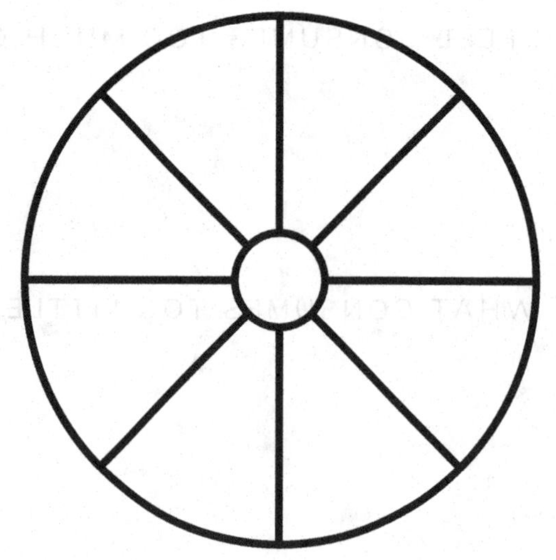

IDEAL TIME
PIE CHART

PLAN TO BRIDGE THE GAP

REAL TIME
PIE CHART

REALIZATIONS ON MAKING SPACE:

RECORD SOME REALIZATIONS YOU HAVE ON MAKING SPACE IN YOUR LIFE AS IT IS CURRENTLY.

MAKE SPACE

Imagine yourself frantically running on a hamster wheel and, as you're reading this, stepping off of it. What a sigh of relief that would be for most people, but a lot of us don't actually want to step off the hamster wheel because we're afraid we will be confronted with our unsightly truths. At least when we are running hard, we don't have to see them. Whereas if we slow down, we may see them and then we'd have to deal with them. So, we just keep up the frantic pace.

I know it's hard, so give yourself some grace here. Just let yourself step off the hamster wheel to go for a walk, read a book, take a nap, or whatever else will allow you to take a breath and regroup. If you're not ready to really see yourself completely right away, that's okay. There's a process that happens when we step back a bit to look at our time and make a little more space for ourselves. Eventually, we enter into a different and better version of ourselves. We become less stressed, less cranky, less tired, less short-fused, more rational, better thinkers, and creators, which makes us more available to others too. This doesn't happen overnight; it happens slowly. As we gift ourselves just a little bit of time back each day, we begin to really see ourselves and identify where we are, how we are doing, and what emotions are popping up.

My encouragement to you would be to let it all come to you naturally. Stepping off the hamster wheel is an act of surrender that has its rewards. It brings a newfound freedom and courage to realize we can, and will, take back some of our time. It's a solid start to feeling more clear-minded and decisive with how we spend our time and what needs to change. Eventually, we will find ourselves in a better space to see what's causing some of the pursuit of distraction or the difficult things in our lives.

A THOUGHT

Turn on the flashlight

Flashlights are meant to cast light on whatever is in the dark. It illuminates reality, so it's often easier to stay in the dark than to face the truth. You might know you need to see what you're really dealing with, but you still might wince as you flip the switch, willing to give anything for it to not go on. Maybe the batteries will be dead! But, alas, it turns on. You slowly open one eye a crack to see what's there...and you realize that what's there, you already know. A lot of what you see has been on repeat in your subconscious mind, which means you haven't noticed that it's been playing in your mind until it's drawn into the light like this.

WHAT SUBCONSCIOUS THOUGHTS HAVE BEEN IN THE DARK THAT I NEED TO BRING INTO THE LIGHT?

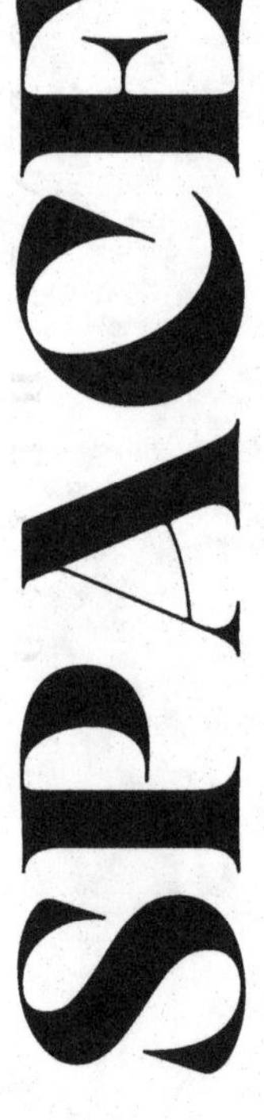

WHAT IMPACT HAVE THOSE SUBCONSCIOUS THOUGHTS BEEN HAVING ON ME?

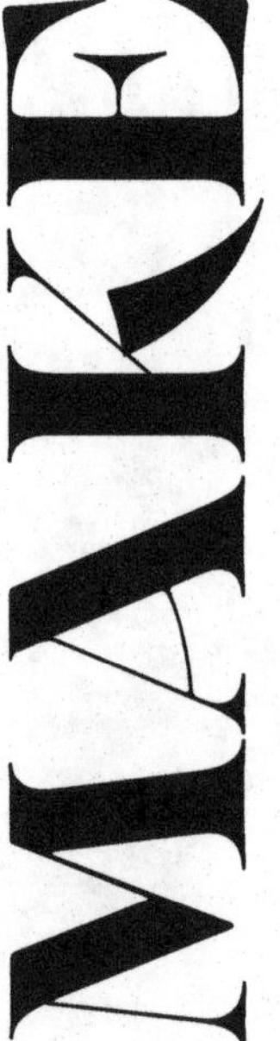

WHAT PREVIOUS WOUNDS MIGHT THOSE INSECURITIES BE COMING FROM?

MAKE SPACE

WHAT STORY HAVE I BELIEVED ABOUT MYSELF THAT ISN'T NECESSARILY TRUE UPON CLOSER EXAMINATION?

WHAT DO I WANT TO REPLACE IT WITH?

"IN MANY CONTEXTS, UNTIL WE LET GO OF WHAT IS NOT GOOD, WE WILL NEVER FIND SOMETHING THAT IS GOOD. THE LESSON: GOOD CANNOT BEGIN UNTIL BAD ENDS."

HENRY CLOUD[6]

FLASHLIGHT REALIZATIONS:

MAKE SPACE

SURRENDER

ONCE WE'VE CLEARED DISTRACTION, MADE SOME TIME, AND TURNED ON THE FLASHLIGHT, WE MAY DISCOVER THAT IT'S OKAY TO WAVE THE WHITE FLAG OF HOLDING ON TO THE WEEDS IN THE WAY.

SOMETIMES, WE SEE THINGS WE DON'T WANT TO SEE WHEN WE TURN ON THE FLASHLIGHT, BUT WE MIGHT REALIZE THE PRISON OF SORTS WE'VE BEEN IN BY HOLDING ONTO THE WEEDS ISN'T WORTH IT. WE DON'T WANT TO BE TRAPPED BY IT ANYMORE.

THIS IS WHEN WE CAN CHOOSE TO SURRENDER OR UPROOT THE WEED IN THE WAY. SOMETIMES, WE CLING TO THINGS AND WE DON'T EVEN KNOW WHY. MAYBE YOU'VE FELT A FEAR OF SOMETHING OR SOMEONE AND IT SEEMED TO KEEP RESURFACING. MAYBE IT'S AN OLD INSECURITY THAT REARS ITS UGLY HEAD AS SIMILAR LIFE SITUATIONS ARISE. THINK ABOUT WHAT IT FELT LIKE WHEN YOU FINALLY LET IT GO THOUGH.

EVEN THOUGH THE OUTCOME WAS UNKNOWN, THE HARDEST PART OF RELEASING SOMETHING IS ACTUALLY MAKING THE DECISION THAT YOU'LL BE FINE WHETHER THE OUTCOME IS FAVORABLE OR NOT. THIS IS SURRENDER.

"GETTING TO THE NEXT LEVEL ALWAYS REQUIRES ENDING SOMETHING, LEAVING IT BEHIND, AND MOVING ON. GROWTH ITSELF DEMANDS THAT WE MOVE ON. WITHOUT THE ABILITY TO END THINGS, PEOPLE STAY STUCK, NEVER BECOMING WHO THEY ARE MEANT TO BE, NEVER ACCOMPLISHING ALL THAT THEIR TALENTS AND ABILITIES SHOULD AFFORD THEM."

HENRY CLOUD[6]

MAKE SPACE

CAN YOU THINK OF A TIME WHEN YOU HELD ONTO SOMETHING LONGER THAN YOU WANTED OR NEEDED TO?

HOW DID IT IMPACT YOU?

IS THERE ANYTHING YOU'RE CURRENTLY HOLDING ONTO THAT YOU KNOW YOU NEED TO SURRENDER?

WHAT LENS ARE YOU VIEWING THINGS THROUGH THAT HAS NEGATIVELY CHANGED THE WAY IN WHICH YOU SEE THINGS?

WHAT NEEDS TO BE DISMANTLED SO THAT YOU CAN START TO VIEW THINGS IN A HEALTHY LIGHT?

SURRENDER REALIZATIONS:

A THOUGHT

"Until you get quiet, you can't know what your heart needs to confess."

Rebekah Lyons[7]

MAKE SPACE

CREATE RHYTHMS

A RHYTHM IS SOMETHING REPEATED; IT'S THE BASELINE THAT YOU CAN ALWAYS RETURN TO.

MAYBE IT'S A NAP ON THE WEEKENDS. MAYBE IT'S FASTING ONCE A WEEK AND FOCUSING ON SOMETHING IN PARTICULAR. EACH TIME YOU FAST, THINK OF THE ONE THING THAT YOU'D LIKE TO HAVE SOME CLARITY ABOUT. MAYBE IT'S WAKING UP EACH MORNING JUST A BIT EARLIER TO HAVE COFFEE IN SILENCE. WHATEVER IT IS FOR YOU, I THINK YOU'LL FIND THAT CREATING RHYTHMS HELPS YOU MAKE SPACE.

WHAT RHYTHMS DO YOU WANT TO MAKE SPACE FOR?

WHAT DO YOU THINK THAT RHYTHM WILL BRING YOU?

ARE THERE ANY RHYTHMS YOU WANT TO GIVE UP?

RHYTHM REALIZATIONS

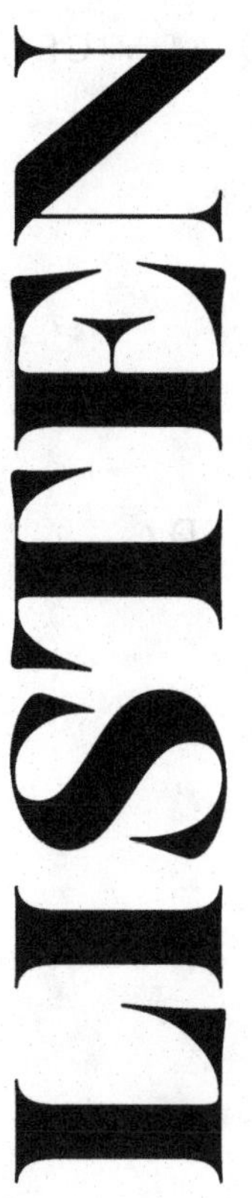

LISTEN.
/'lisn/
verb
give one's attention to a sound.

I've found that after making some space, thoughts and words flood in—in a good way. I can hear that still, small voice inside of me that sets me on course. It grounds me and comforts me as I lead the way through this messy life. Listening in this way has been such a gift to me, and I know it can be for you too.

After we clear the room, uproot the weeds in the way, and turn on the flashlight, we get to enjoy the rewards that come from it. We won't feel the need to overcompensate, overachieve, talk over others to be heard, or try to prove ourselves. We can just be right where we are, in a posture to listen to ourselves and others.

DON'T FOCUS ENERGY ON FIGHTING OR CRAFTING A RESPONSE

WHERE OR WHEN DO I FIND MYSELF GETTING DEFENSIVE?

ARE THERE REPEATED PATTERNS OR RELATIONSHIPS THAT TRIGGER ME?

ARE THERE PLACES WHERE I GIVE UNSOLICITED ADVICE?

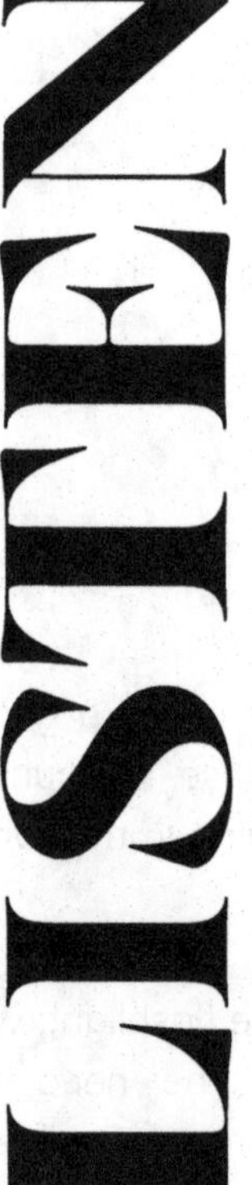

WHAT WOULD HAPPEN IF I PURELY LISTENED?

ARE THERE PEOPLE IN MY LIFE THAT I AM TRYING TO CHANGE?

WHAT WOULD HAPPEN IF I STOPPED?

ARE THERE ANY ACTIONS I WANT TO TAKE OR CHANGES I WANT TO MAKE IN LIGHT OF ANSWERING THESE QUESTIONS?

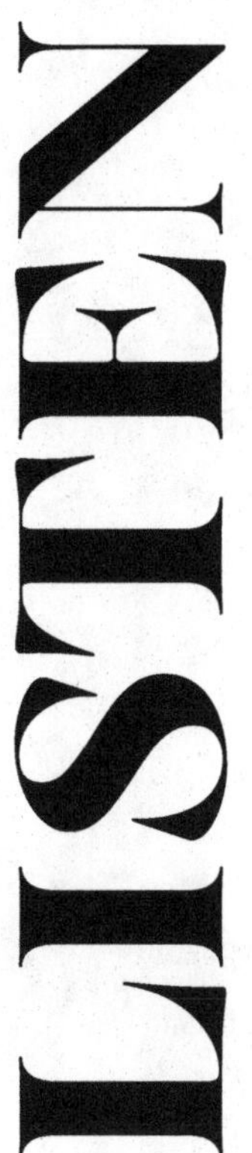

SHOW INTEREST

HAVE YOU EVER BEEN WITH SOMEONE WHO DIDN'T ASK YOU ONE QUESTION ABOUT YOURSELF? YOU TALKED ABOUT THE WEATHER, THEMSELVES, AND EVERYTHING OTHER THAN YOURSELF. WHEN I FIND MYSELF IN THOSE ONE-SIDED INTERACTIONS, I TEND TO FEEL UNNOTICED. QUESTIONS COMMUNICATE INTEREST, SO WHEN WE FEEL LIKE SOMEONE HAS AN INTEREST IN US, WE FEEL VALUED.

WHAT WAS A TIME FOR ME THAT I EXPERIENCED A ONE SIDED CONVERSATION?

HOW DID IT MAKE ME FEEL?

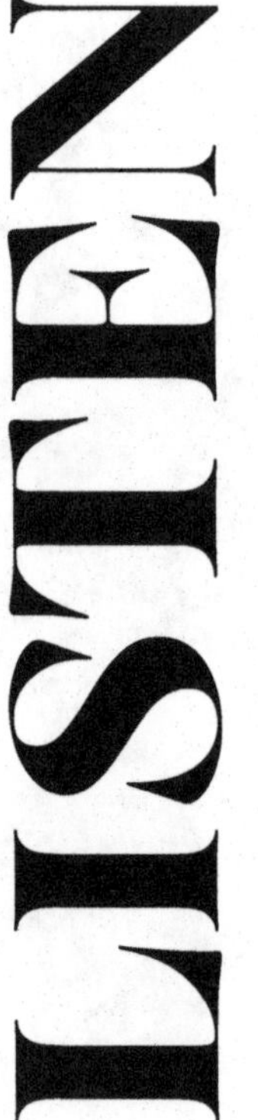

ARE THERE RELATIONSHIPS THAT I CONTINUOUSLY SEE THIS HAPPENING?

CAN YOU THINK OF A TIME WHEN EITHER ANSWERING GOOD QUESTIONS FROM SOMEONE ELSE HELPED YOU UNCOVER SOME REALIZATIONS ABOUT SOMETHING THAT LED TO GROWTH OR CHANGE OR YOU ASKED A GOOD QUESTION AND IT HELPED THE PERSON ANSWERING PROCESS SOMETHING MEANINGFUL?

IN YOUR RELATIONSHIPS, DO YOU TEND TO SHOW INTEREST IN OTHERS?

WHAT SHIFTS DO YOU MAKE TO MAKE IN LIGHT OF YOUR DISCOVERIES HERE?

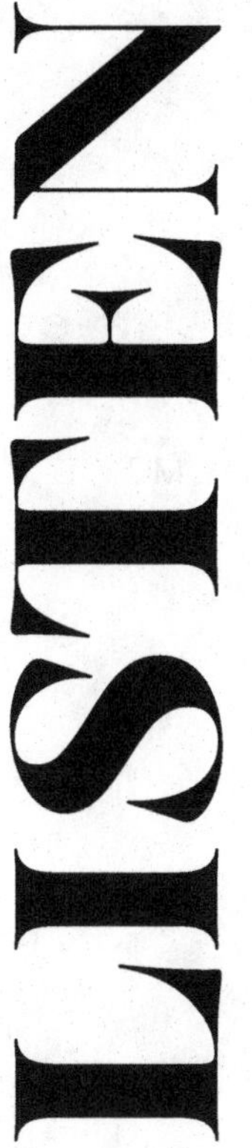

CLARIFY WHAT THEY WANT FROM YOU

CONVERSATIONS ARE OFTEN TRANSACTIONAL IN NATURE, BUT WE MAY MISS OUT ON WHAT IS ACTUALLY BEING ASKED IF WE DON'T LISTEN CAREFULLY OR FULLY UNDERSTAND THEIR NEEDS. IF YOU MISS THIS, GET CLARITY ON WHAT THEY ACTUALLY NEED FROM YOU. WE SOMETIMES COMPLETELY MISINTERPRET WHAT THE OTHER PERSON IS ASKING FOR BECAUSE WE EITHER AREN'T LISTENING CAREFULLY OR WE DON'T UNDERSTAND THEIR REAL NEED. UNDERSTANDING WHAT OTHERS WANT FROM YOU WILL HELP YOU LISTEN BETTER. DO THEY WANT TO VENT? DO THEY WANT HELP FIGURING OUT WHAT TO DO? ASKING QUESTIONS SUCH AS "HOW CAN I BEST HELP YOU?" WILL BRING CLARIFICATION.

IS THERE A PERSON OR REPEATED PATTERN IN YOUR LIFE THAT YOU'RE UNSURE ON WHAT THEY'RE LOOKING FOR FROM YOU?

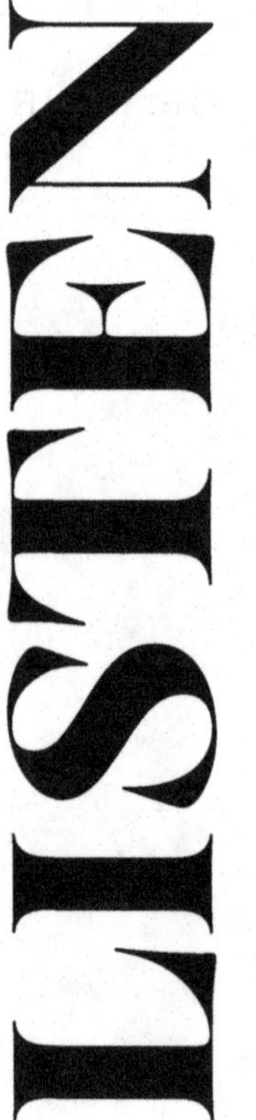

WHAT DO YOU FEEL WHEN YOU'RE WITH THEM?

HAVE YOU ASKED THEM HOW YOU CAN BEST HELP THEM OR WHAT THEY MIGHT BE LOOKING FOR FROM YOU? (SUPPORT, COMFORT, ADVICE)

ARE THERE ANY ASSUMPTIONS THAT YOU'VE MADE ABOUT YOURSELF OR THEM BECAUSE OF A LACK OF CLARITY ON WHAT THEY MIGHT BE WANTING FROM YOU?

HAVE YOU ASKED THEM HOW YOU CAN BEST HELP THEM OR WHAT THEY MIGHT BE LOOKING FOR FROM YOU? (SUPPORT, COMFORT, ADVICE)

ARE THERE ANY ASSUMPTIONS THAT YOU'VE MADE ABOUT YOURSELF OR THEM BECAUSE OF A LACK OF CLARITY ON WHAT THEY MIGHT BE WANTING FROM YOU?

LISTEN

GET IN THE BOAT WITH THEM

NO ONE WANTS TO FEEL ALONE IN ANYTHING. IT'S PRETTY HARD TO FEEL LIKE THERE AREN'T PEOPLE OUT THERE WHO RESONATE WITH WHAT YOU'RE FEELING. ISOLATION CREEPS IN, AND THEN DARKNESS CAN GRAB A FOOTHOLD. THAT FOOTHOLD CAN MAKE US BELIEVE LIES ABOUT OURSELVES AND OTHERS, KEEPING US TRAPPED OR STUCK IN ISOLATION.

WE NEED TO FIGHT AGAINST PEOPLE FEELING ALONE, UNSEEN, UNKNOWN, OR UNHEARD. CAN YOU IMAGINE HOW OUR WORLD WOULD CHANGE? IT WOULD REVERSE OLD WOUNDS, HEAL UP HEARTS, CHANGE CONVERSATIONS, TAKE DOWN DEFENSIVENESS, AND SO MUCH MORE. IN OUR DIVISIVE, POLARIZED CULTURE, THIS IS THE BEGINNING OF THE ANSWER. EVERYONE CAN PRACTICE THIS, NO ONE IS EXCLUDED. WE ALL HAVE THE OPPORTUNITY TO GO A LITTLE DEEPER, WADE INTO THE WATER, AND GET IN THE BOAT WITH THE PEOPLE IN OUR LIVES.

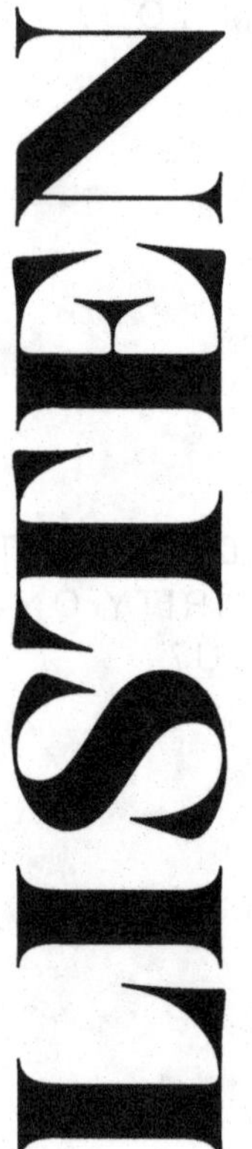

HOWEVER, OUR OWN SELVES OFTEN PREVENT US FROM DOING THIS AS WE'RE PRIMARILY FOCUSED ON OUR OWN WANTS AND NEEDS. WHEN WE START STEPPING INTO THE BOAT WITH OTHERS, WE GAIN PERSPECTIVE, UNDERSTANDING, CONNECTEDNESS, AND PURPOSE. IMAGINE YOURSELF CLIMBING INTO YOUR FRIEND, COWORKER, OR SIGNIFICANT OTHER'S BOAT. WHAT'S IT LIKE? WHAT DO THEY WRESTLE WITH? WHAT DO THEY CELEBRATE? YOU CAN'T SOLVE THEIR PROBLEMS (NOR SHOULD YOU), CHANGE OUTCOMES, OR CHANGE THEM, BUT YOU CAN ALWAYS GET IN THE BOAT WITH THEM.

WHO IS COMING TO MIND RIGHT NOW THAT YOU CAN "GET IN THE BOAT" WITH?

WHERE ARE YOU FEELING ALONE IN YOUR LIFE?

HOW CAN YOU ASK/GET SUPPORT?

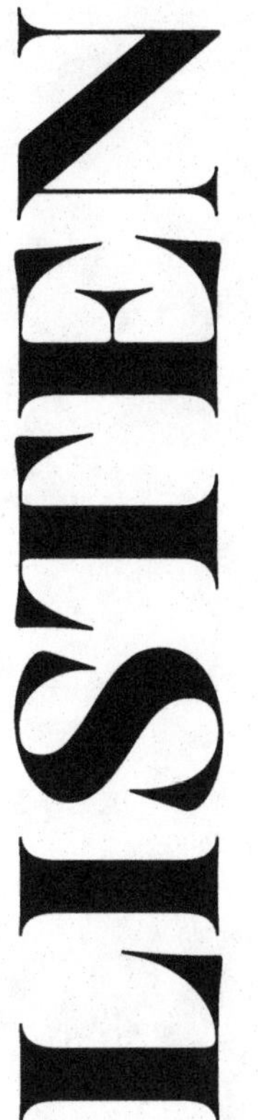

WHAT KEEPS YOU FROM GETTING THE SUPPORT YOU NEED?

WHAT KEEPS YOU FROM "GETTING IN THE BOAT" WITH OTHERS?

A THOUGHT

Cultivate the ability to listen to yourself.

It's a gift that you can give to yourself! Listening to ourselves is the foundation for learning to listen to others. Listening to ourselves is grounded in becoming more self-aware.

AN OPPORTUNITY

Take a day where you focus on listening to your responses in conversations throughout the day.

Think about how you responded to each situation and person you interacted with that day.

LISTEN FOR A DAY REFLECTIONS

WHAT TRIGGERS CAME UP FOR YOU?

WHAT RESPONSES FELT DEFENSIVE OR LIKE YOU WERE TRYING TO PROVE YOURSELF?

WHAT RESPONSES FELT WISE OR RIGHT ON POINT?

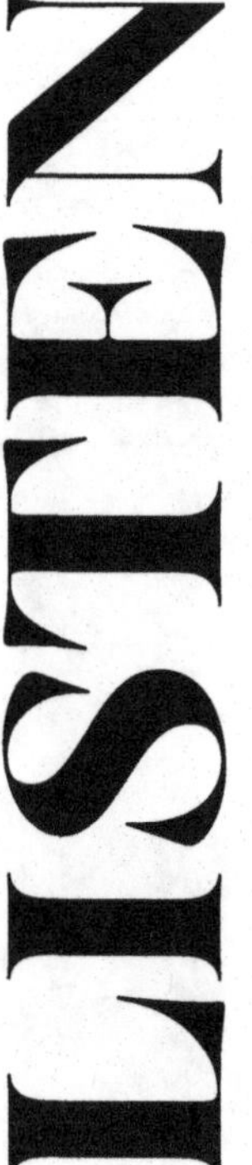

WHAT BLIND SPOTS CAN YOU IDENTIFY AS A RESULT OF LISTENING TO YOURSELF IN CONVERSATION?

DID YOU SEE PEOPLES' EYES BEGIN TO DRIFT OFF AS YOU TALKED TOO LONG ABOUT YOURSELF OR A TOPIC?

DID YOU SEE PEOPLES' EXPRESSIONS CHANGE IN A NEGATIVE WAY WHILE YOU WERE TALKING?

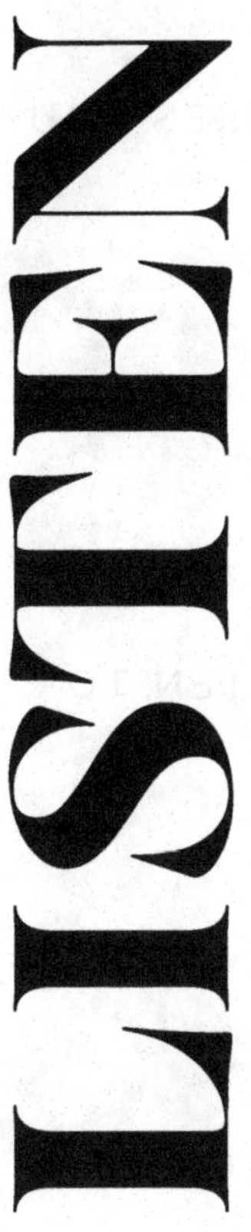

THIS IS WHERE YOU CAN, AND SHOULD, ALSO CONSIDER ASKING FOR FEEDBACK ABOUT YOU AS A COMMUNICATOR FROM A TRUSTED FRIEND. YOU MAY BE THINKING THAT THEIR EXPRESSIONS ARE SAYING SOMETHING THAT THEY'RE NOT BASED ON INTERNAL MESSAGES FROM PREVIOUS WOUNDS. WHEN THIS HAPPENS, YOUR LENS MAY NOT BE ACCURATE, WHICH CAN CAUSE US TO MAKE A LOT OF ASSUMPTIONS ABOUT HOW AND WHY PEOPLE ARE RESPONDING TO US AS THEY ARE. VERIFYING THESE PERCEPTIONS OF YOURSELF IN TRUSTED CIRCLES IS EXTREMELY IMPORTANT BECAUSE IT'S PART OF THE PROCESS OF GETTING OUT OF YOUR OWN WAY SO THAT YOU CAN BE FREE TO HEAR OTHERS.

CULTIVATE THE ABILITY TO LISTEN TO OTHERS

LISTENING IS HARD WORK, AND IT TAKES PRACTICE TO PERFECT IT. HERE ARE SOME TIPS FOR CULTIVATING THE ABILITY TO DO IT WELL:

REPEAT BACK WHAT THEY'VE SAID
VISUALIZE THEIR SITUATION
ALLOW FOR SILENCES AND PAUSES
ASK QUESTIONS WITH MOTIVES OR BIAS

WHO DO YOU WANT TO SPEND TIME LISTENING TO IN YOUR LIFE?

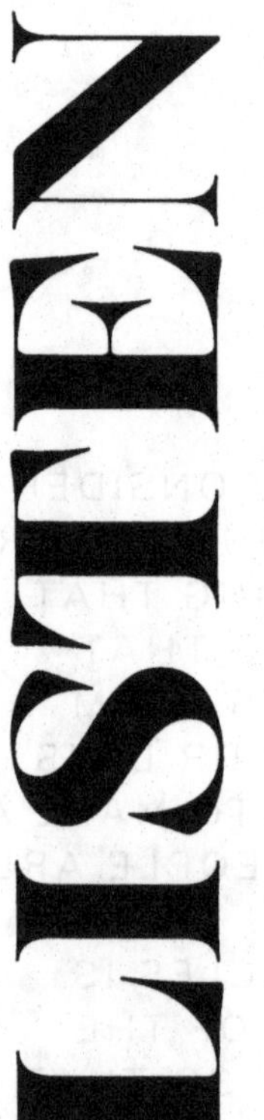

AS YOU VISUALIZE THEIR SITUATION, WHAT STRIKES YOU?

HOW WOULD THIS CHANGE THE WAY YOU LISTEN TO THEM?

DO YOU ALLOW FOR SILENCES AND PAUSES IN YOUR CONVERSATIONS? WHY OR WHY NOT?

WHAT WOULD ALLOWING FOR SOME MORE SILENCE ALLOW SPACE FOR?

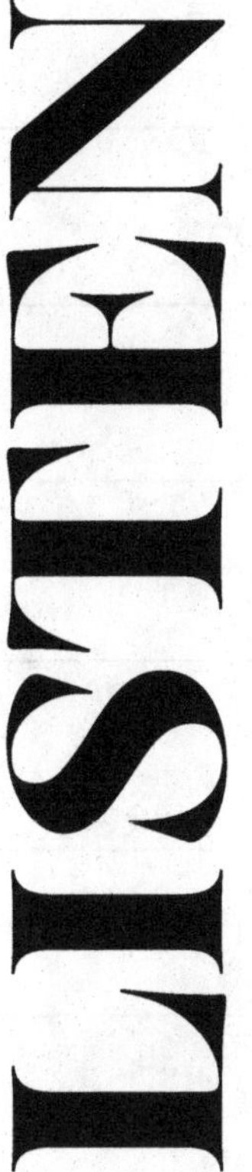

WHAT MIGHT PREVENT YOU FROM LISTENING WELL TO OTHERS?

REALIZATIONS ON LISTENING

UNDERSTAND

LISTENING LEADS TO UNDERSTANDING.

WE CAN HEAR THINGS ALL DAY LONG BUT NOT TRANSLATE THEM TO BE ABLE TO UNDERSTAND THEM. WHEN WE MISS THIS STEP, WE CAN FALL SHORT OF EXPERIENCING LIFE TO THE FULLEST. ULTIMATELY, WE CAN MISS THE MEANING BEHIND THE MOMENTS. IF WE UNDERSTAND OURSELVES AND OTHERS MORE DEEPLY, WE CAN EXPERIENCE THE CONNECTEDNESS THAT MAKES US THRIVE.

WHO ARE THOSE IN YOUR LIFE THAT YOU RELATE TO EASILY? IS IT EASIER TO UNDERSTAND THEM?

ARE THERE THOSE THAT YOU CAN'T RELATE TO BUT STILL UNDERSTAND?

WHY DO YOU THINK YOU'RE ABLE TO UNDERSTAND THEM?

WHO IN YOUR LIFE CAN YOU NOT UNDERSTAND OR RELATE TO? WHY IS THAT?

UNDERSTAND

REFLECT BACK ON YOUR TIME WITH THEM.

IT'S IN THE REFLECTING THAT WE HAVE AN OPPORTUNITY TO SLOW DOWN A BIT, AND THINK ABOUT WHAT THEY WERE REALLY SAYING.

CHALLENGE YOURSELF TO WRITE SOME NOTES ABOUT WHAT YOU SAW OR HEARD FROM THEM IN YOUR CONVERSATION.

THAT NOTE WILL INFLUENCE HOW YOU LOOK AT THEM, INTERACT WITH THEM, AND CONDUCT YOURSELF AROUND THEM. THIS EXERCISE ISN'T NECESSARILY MEANT TO BE SHARED WITH THEM; IT'S FOR YOUR PERSONAL REFLECTION AND UNDERSTANDING, SO THEY MIGHT NEVER BE ABLE TO PUT THEIR FINGER ON WHAT EXACTLY HAS DEEPENED YOUR UNDERSTANDING OF THEM, BUT THEY'LL FEEL IT. IN TURN, THEY WILL LIKELY OPEN THE DOOR A LITTLE WIDER FOR MORE CONVERSATION BECAUSE WHEN PEOPLE FEEL UNDERSTOOD, THEY FEEL SAFE.

HOW DO I WANT TO PRACTICE REFLECTING ON MY TIME WITH OTHERS?

UNDERSTAND

ACCEPT THAT YOU WILL NEVER FULLY KNOW THEM.

WE'LL NEVER KNOW SOMEONE ELSE FULLY BECAUSE WE ARE SO MULTIFACETED AND COMPLEX, AND WE ARE ALWAYS CHANGING. WE CAN'T KNOW EVERY SINGLE THOUGHT, FEELING, REACTION, DECISION, OR DESIRE OF SOMEONE ELSE: IT'S SIMPLY IMPOSSIBLE. THE NUMBER OF THOUGHTS AND FEELINGS THAT PASS THROUGH OUR BRAINS EACH DAY IS ASTOUNDING, AND WHEN WE THINK ABOUT THAT IN COMPARISON TO THE NUMBER OF THEM THAT WE SHARE WITH OTHERS, IT'S ONLY A FRACTION. ONLY GOD KNOWS EVERYTHING ABOUT US.

REMEMBER THIS— WE CAN KNOW PEOPLE OR TRY TO CHANGE PEOPLE, SO ALWAYS GO WITH KNOWING THEM.

UNDERSTAND

AS I THINK ABOUT MYSELF, WHO DO I MAKE MYSELF KNOWN TO THE MOST? WHY?

WHO DO I WANT TO MAKE MYSELF KNOWN TO MORE? WHY?

HOW CAN I KNOW MYSELF MORE?

WHAT DOES GOD WANT TO REVEAL TO ME ABOUT MYSELF?

ARE THERE ANY AREAS WHERE I'M TRYING TO CHANGE PEOPLE RATHER THAN SIMPLY KNOW THEM?

UNDERSTAND

IF YOU GET STUCK, LISTEN SOME MORE.

CAN YOU THINK OF A TIME WHERE YOU GOT STUCK IN THE UNDERSTANDING PHASE? WHERE YOU JUST COULDN'T GET TO THAT PLACE OF SEEING, HEARING, AND KNOWING SOMEONE. OLD WOUNDS, INSECURITIES, OR PREVIOUS PATTERNS IN A RELATIONSHIP FEEL AS IF THEY WERE ACTING AS A BLOCK TO TAKING IN ANYTHING THE OTHER PERSON HAD TO SAY. YOU FEEL ANGRY, HURT, DEPRESSED, OR FAILED BECAUSE OF ATTEMPTS TO WORK IT OUT. AFTER VENTING OR PROCESSING YOUR WEEDS IN THE WAY, YOU CAN ALWAYS GO BACK TO LISTENING. TIME AND TIME AGAIN, THIS IS CENTRAL TO UNDERSTANDING, AND YOU CAN RETURN TO AS MANY TIMES AS NEEDED. A RETURN TO LISTENING WILL POSITION YOU TO IDENTIFY WHAT IS BEING SAID AND NOT SAID BY YOURSELF AND WITH OTHERS. IT GIVES YOU GROUNDS FOR A RESET AND REFRESHES YOU TO BE ABLE TO CONTINUE MOVING FORWARD IN A NEW AND BETTER WAY.

WHAT SITUATIONS OR RELATIONSHIPS DO YOU FEEL STUCK IN THE UNDERSTANDING PHASE?

IS THERE AN OLD WOUND, INSECURITY, OR PREVIOUS PATTERN THAT MAY BE CONTRIBUTING TO BEING STUCK?

IN LIGHT OF YOUR DISCOVERIES HERE, IS THERE ANYTHING YOU WANT TO CLARIFY OR VERIFY WITH YOURSELF, A PARTICULAR SITUATION, OR RELATIONSHIP?

REALIZATIONS ON UNDERSTANDING

A THOUGHT

As we've looked at the Seen, Known, and Heard framework so far, we see that each step builds upon each other.

When we make space, we clear the way for ourselves and others to process all that life brings our way.

It sets us up to listen with ears to hear with clarity rather than the fogginess that can come from our weeds in the way.

As we listen more clearly, our understanding improves.

We'll be more discerning and experience the fullness that comes from reflection.

The last part of the framework can be the most rewarding, and that is the ability to give and receive communication.

COMMUNICATE

COMMUNICATE.
/kəˈmyo͞onəˌkāt/
verb
share or exchange information, news, or ideas.

After we've listened (which itself is a form of communication), we have the chance to communicate back to others. This includes letting them know that we see them, that we've taken the time to understand what life looks like from their perspective, that we've truly "digested" what they've shared, and that we are tracking with them.

Here are a few tangible ways we can practice letting others know that we're with them:

Know their name
Look them in the eyes
Take down your defenses
Repeat back what they said
Notice the little things
Communicate in love

COMMUNICATE

KNOW THEIR NAME.

CAREER COACH JOYCE E. A. RUSSELL EXPLAINS WHY IT'S SO IMPORTANT TO USE PEOPLE'S NAMES.

A PERSON'S NAME IS THE GREATEST CONNECTION TO THEIR OWN IDENTITY AND INDIVIDUALITY. SOME MIGHT SAY IT IS THE MOST IMPORTANT WORD IN THE WORLD TO THAT PERSON. IT IS THE ONE WAY WE CAN EASILY GET SOMEONE'S ATTENTION. IT IS A SIGN OF COURTESY AND A WAY OF RECOGNIZING THEM. WHEN SOMEONE REMEMBERS OUR NAME AFTER MEETING US, WE FEEL RESPECTED AND MORE IMPORTANT. IT MAKES A POSITIVE AND LASTING IMPRESSION ON US.[8]

WHAT DOES MY NAME MEAN TO ME?

HOW DO I RESPOND DIFFERENTLY WHEN SOMEONE KNOWS AND USES MY NAME?

HOW CAN I DO THAT FOR OTHERS?

COMMUNICATE

LOOK THEM IN THE EYES.

PEOPLE PAY MORE ATTENTION TO ONE ANOTHER WHEN THEY KNOW THE OTHER PERSON IS FOCUSED ON THEM. I DON'T KNOW ABOUT YOU, BUT I'M MUCH MORE APT TO PAY ATTENTION IF SOMEONE IS SITTING IN FRONT OF ME, MAKING EYE CONTACT, WITHOUT ANY DISTRACTIONS CAPTURING THEIR GAZE. EYE CONTACT IS A SIMPLE THING THAT WE ALL CAN DO WHEN TALKING TO OTHERS. IT COMMUNICATES THAT WE'RE PRESENT AND TAKING THE TIME TO SEE, KNOW, AND HEAR THEM. IT FOSTERS MEANINGFUL CONNECTION AND CREATES MOMENTS THAT STICK WITH US.

THINK OF A MEMORY WITH SOMEONE THAT STICKS IN YOUR MIND. IF YOU CAN REMEMBER THE SETTING AND THE EXCHANGE YOU SHARED, I'D BET THAT EYE CONTACT WAS A PART OF THAT MOMENT. WE CAN CREATE THE SAME FOR OTHERS WHEN WE OFFER THEM EYE CONTACT.

WHO IN MY LIFE IS GOOD AT LOOKING ME IN THE EYES WHEN THEY TALK TO ME?

HOW DOES THAT MAKE ME FEEL?

COMMUNICATE

WHERE AM I STRONG IN MAKING EYE CONTACT WITH OTHERS?

ARE THERE SITUATIONS WHERE I AVOID EYE CONTACT? WHY IS THAT?

ARE THERE ANY CHANGES I WANT TO MAKE IN LIGHT OF THIS?

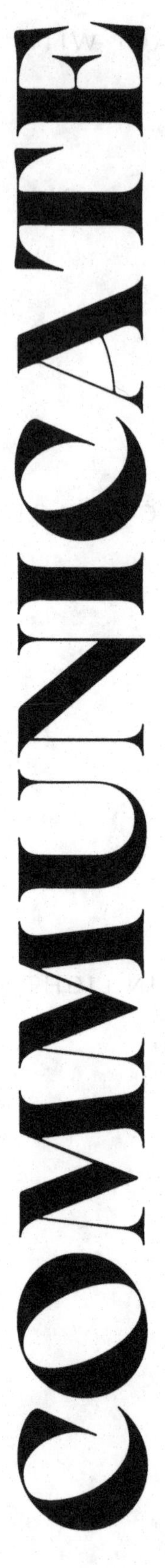

TAKE DOWN YOUR DEFENSES.

PAY ATTENTION TO YOUR POSTURE. POSTURE CAN REFLECT YOUR DISPOSITION. IT NONVERBALLY COMMUNICATES YOUR VIEWS ABOUT YOURSELF OR HOW YOU MIGHT BE FEELING ABOUT THE PEOPLE IN FRONT OF YOU. YOUR POSTURE COMMUNICATES YOUR THOUGHTS. IT REPRESENTS HOW YOU FEEL ABOUT YOURSELF AND HOW YOU'RE FEELING ABOUT OTHERS. UNCROSS YOUR ARMS, LEAN IN, AND BE STILL AS YOU LISTEN TO WHOEVER IS IN FRONT OF YOU. WE CAN GIVE OTHERS THAT GIFT EVERY DAY—SHOWING THEM WITH OUR BODY LANGUAGE THAT WE'RE PRESENT.

WHEN YOU THINK ABOUT HOW YOU COMMUNICATE WITH THOSE AROUND YOU, CAN YOU THINK OF CERTAIN SITUATIONS IN WHICH YOU LEAN IN BECAUSE YOU FEEL SAFE OR INTERESTED IN WHAT THAT PERSON HAS TO SAY?

NOW THINK OF A TIME WHEN YOU FELT DEFENSIVE, UNSURE, OR HESITANT TO TRUST. WHAT WAS YOUR PHYSICAL RESPONSE?

WHAT IS THIS REVEALING TO YOU ABOUT YOUR RELATIONSHIPS?

ARE THERE ANY CHANGES YOU WANT TO MAKE IN LIGHT OF YOUR DISCOVERIES OR ANYTHING THAT YOU'VE SIMPLY BECOME AWARE OF?

COMMUNICATE

REPEAT BACK WHAT THEY SAID.

YOU DON'T HAVE TO REPEAT EVERY WORD THEY SAY TO PROVE YOU'RE LISTENING AND ENGAGED, BUT IT DOES HELP TO REPEAT THE IMPORTANT PARTS OF THE CONVERSATION OR TO ASK FOR FURTHER EXPLANATION ABOUT A PARTICULAR STATEMENT THEY MADE. WE VALIDATE THEIR WORDS WHILE SQUASHING ANY JUDGMENTS OR ASSUMPTIONS WE MAY MAKE BY NOT ASKING FOR CLARIFICATION.

HAS ANYONE EVER REPEATED BACK PART OF WHAT YOU SAID, AND IT WASN'T REALLY WHAT YOU MEANT? WHEN WAS THIS?

MAYBE WHEN YOU HEARD IT BACK, THE WORDS WERE ACCURATE, BUT YOU REALIZED YOU HADN'T EXPLAINED YOURSELF WELL OR EVEN PROCESSED THE TOPIC YOU ARE DISCUSSING WELL?

IS THERE ANYONE IN YOUR LIFE WHO CLARIFIES WHAT YOU'RE SAYING WELL?

ARE THERE ANY REALIZATIONS THAT YOU WANT TO TAKE WITH YOU IN LIGHT OF YOUR DISCOVERIES HERE?

COMMUNICATE

NOTICE THE LITTLE THINGS.

SOMETIMES, THE LITTLE THINGS ARE THE BIG THINGS. HAVE YOU EVER BEEN IN CONVERSATION WITH SOMEONE AND THEY MENTIONED SOMETHING YOU SAID PREVIOUSLY OR SOMETHING YOU DID OR WORE? AT THAT MOMENT, I'M GUESSING YOU FELT NOTICED.

BEING NOTICED MAKES US FEEL VALUED, AND IT'S SOMETHING THAT WE CAN ALL DO. MAKE MENTAL NOTES WHEN YOU COME AWAY FROM A CONVERSATION. WHAT DO YOU WANT TO REMEMBER ABOUT THAT CONVERSATION? WHAT DID YOU SEE? REMEMBER THE LITTLE THINGS—PARTICULARLY THE GOOD THINGS—BECAUSE THEY CAN GO A LONG WAY IN FOSTERING MEANINGFUL CONNECTIONS WITH OTHERS.

WHAT "LITTLE THINGS" MAKE YOU FEEL NOTICED?

WHO DOES THIS IN YOUR LIFE?

COMMUNICATE

HOW CAN YOU NOTICE YOURSELF IN THE SMALL WAYS THAT MATTER TO YOU?

CAN YOU GIVE YOURSELF WHAT YOU NEED HERE?

HOW CAN YOU DO THIS FOR THOSE AROUND YOU?

COMMUNICATE

TELL THEM.

THINK ABOUT A TIME WHEN A FRIEND CALLED OUT SOMETHING THEY SAW IN YOU, AND IT WAS FROM A GENUINE PLACE. THERE WERE NO ULTERIOR MOTIVES OR MANIPULATION—JUST TRUTH. HOW REFRESHING AND LIFE-GIVING WERE THOSE WORDS TO YOU? HAVE YOU HELD ONTO THEM, SAVED THEM IN A SCREENSHOT, OR THOUGHT OF THEM OFTEN WHEN YOU NEEDED THEM? I KNOW I HAVE BECAUSE THEY ENCOURAGE ME WHEN I FEEL DOWN OR UNCERTAIN OF WHETHER WHAT I'M DOING OR FEELING MAKES A DIFFERENCE. WORDS CAN SPEAK LIFE OR DEATH; IT'S OUR CHOICE IN HOW WE USE THEM AND RECEIVE THEM.

WHEN HAS THIS HAPPENED TO ME?

WHAT DID IT MEAN TO ME?

COMMUNICATE

WHAT WERE THE WORDS SPOKEN TO ME?

HOW DID THAT ENCOURAGE ME/WHAT CAME AS A RESULT OF THAT?

HOW DO I WANT TO DO THIS FOR MYSELF AND OTHERS MOVING FORWARD?

COMMUNICATE

DON'T JUMP TO OFFER ADVICE.

CAN YOU THINK OF A TIME WHEN SOMEONE JUMPED IN QUICKLY TO TELL YOU WHAT YOU SHOULD OR COULD DO IN A PARTICULAR SITUATION YOU WERE SHARING WITH THEM?

HOW DID THAT MAKE YOU FEEL?

WHAT DID YOU WANT INSTEAD?

ARE THERE SCENARIOS WHERE YOU FIND YOURSELF GIVING UNSOLICITED ADVICE?

WHAT SHIFTS DO YOU WANT TO MAKE IN LIGHT OF HOW YOU RECEIVE FROM OTHERS/WHAT YOU GIVE TO OTHERS IN LIGHT OF YOUR DISCOVERIES HERE?

COMMUNICATE

COMMUNICATE IN LOVE.

MUSIC CAN BE APPRECIATED, BUT ONLY IF IT'S IN TUNE, ON KEY, AND IN SYNC. IF IT'S NOT, WE WANT IT TO STOP. WE DON'T WANT TO HEAR IT. LIKEWISE, COMMUNICATION, WITHOUT A BASE OF LOVE, IS MUCH THE SAME. IT CAN'T BE RECEIVED OR HEARD BECAUSE THE MOTIVE ISN'T PURE AND SELFLESS.

CAN I THINK OF A TIME OR PERSON THAT COMMUNICATES WITH A BASE OF LOVE?

WHAT IS IT ABOUT THEIR COMMUNICATION THAT CONFIRMS THIS TO ME?

HOW DO I COMMUNICATE WITH OTHERS?

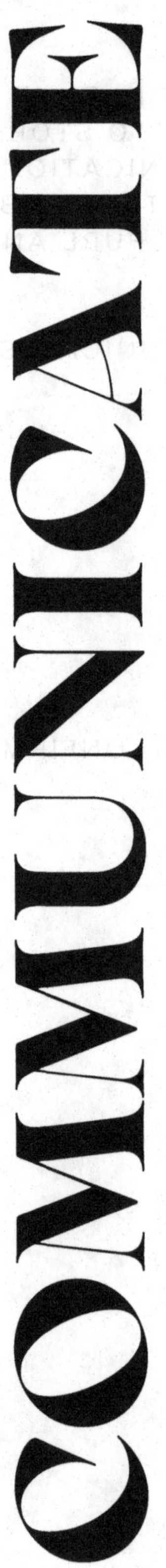

WHAT DO I WANT TO CONTINUE DOING IN REGARDS TO HOW I COMMUNICATE WITH OTHERS?

WHAT DO I WANT TO SHIFT?

WHAT INTERNAL SHIFTS NEED TO HAPPEN IN ME TO MAKE THAT POSSIBLE?

COMMUNICATION REALIZATIONS

How it Changes Everything

MAKE SPACE
LISTEN
UNDERSTAND
COMMUNICATE

As we near the end of our time together, I want to give you a place to think about what your life would look like as you see, know, and hear others more and how it could possibly change things for you. So, let's review the benefits of incorporating this framework into your daily life.

MAKE SPACE

You've made space by clearing out some of your "weeds in the way".

You've surrendered some things you might have been holding onto, realizing they were imprisoning you.

You've recognized some things that might be hijacking your time and replaced them with some rhythms that will fill you up instead of deplete you.

What is your next making space step?

LISTEN

You don't feel the need to spend your energy crafting a response toward others, but instead lean in to ask questions.

You clarify what they might be looking for from you and are able to "get in the boat" with them.

You've cultivated the ability to listen to yourself and others. A quiet contentment emerges.

What is your next listening step?

UNDERSTAND

As you're with yourself and others, you notice yourself reflecting back on your time with them, and things start coming to mind. You take note of them and learn that communication is so much more than words.

You're realizing incredible things through the process of starting to translate what you hear being said.

You know that you can always go back to listening more if you get stuck, and you feel a grace and a freedom in knowing that you'll never fully know each human on the planet.

What is your next understanding step?

COMMUNICATE

You find more joy in daily life: noticing peoples' names, looking them in the eyes, and feeling free from putting up defenses.

As you realize you aren't in control of anybody else but yourself, a new freedom to communicate with clarity comes.

Noticing the little things, telling them what you see in them, and not jumping to offer advice serves you well.

You leave conversations with less regret and experience a fullness that comes with more meaningful communication throughout your days.

What is your next communication step?

THE PEOPLE IN YOUR LIFE

As we've talked about, being seen, known, and heard is all about people. No AI or technology can replace the power of human-to-human connection and the seemingly intangible but powerful culture that shifts neighborhoods, workplaces, schools, governments, families, and friendships. This cannot and should not be underestimated. No amount of benchmarks can measure the power of this framework.

Let's look together at the people in your life for a few minutes and envision what could be as you engage with the framework:

THE PEOPLE IN YOUR LIFE

Neighbors

The people you encounter everyday know that they're valued just by the way you interact with them. You start to see them beyond the hello, and you find your life fuller of little moments of connection throughout the day that create joy.

Coworkers

Those coworkers that were so irritating to you just a bit ago don't get under your skin as much as they used to. It's like you've turned the wheel on the end of the kaleidoscope and see them from a different angle now. They might not have changed, but you have. You've started to notice and understand where some of their patterns might come from, and you find yourself responding differently because of it.

Customers

As a business owner, you've stopped the frantic pace for just a day, long enough to really see, hear, and know your customer. It's completely changed your perspective, and you don't feel the need to overcompensate with doing extra tasks that aren't contributing to the heart of the business. You have clarity on your next steps and priorities as a result of this work, and you feel the tension and anxiety over the future of the business dissipate.

THE PEOPLE IN YOUR LIFE

Family

The family members that used to trigger you don't as much anymore. Sure, you still have moments where you notice your blood pressure rising, but you catch it. You recognize the pattern, understand its roots, and check in with yourself to think about responding differently. You find that the connections are more meaningful, and they, whether they realize it or not, have started to let their normal defenses down a bit because they feel seen, known, and heard.

Friends

You recognize the different levels of friendship and appreciate them for how they each play an integral role in your life, some in seemingly small ways and others in larger ways. Depending on the season of life, these roles tend to shift around, and you recognize and value that shift. You appreciate each person for where they are, and you enjoy walking with them through life.

THE PEOPLE IN YOUR LIFE

Public Figures

You see that it's as difficult a time as any to be a public figure in any space and seek to understand and recognize a heightened awareness to influences around them that are shifting and shaping their behaviors and statements. It helps you as you navigate through the curation of the information that you're taking in.

Ourselves

You've taken the time to see, know, and hear yourself a bit more. You find that you're more aware of the things that trigger you and the things that you like and don't like. It's almost like you're watching yourself as you move through the days. You're having realizations and learning to enjoy who you are. You find less of a need to overcompensate, explain, or justify everything you're doing.

PEOPLE IN YOUR LIFE REALIZATIONS

THE CHARGE AS YOU GO FORWARD

As I seek to sum up this journey we've walked through together, I'm reminded that nothing comes without sacrifice. Seeing, knowing, and hearing yourself and others definitely requires the sacrifice of time, but it's some of the best time you'll ever spend. It changes everything, and the person it may change the most is you.

Everywhere I went over the last several years, I seemed to recognize the need for people to see, know, and hear themselves and others. I'm grateful for this transformation because it has led to a more fulfilling, meaningful life. My hope is that it will do the same for you.

People will always remember who you were to them. The kind of neighbor, client, friend, parent, and human you are to those around you will have a lasting influence because you impact people whether you want to or not. We are the leaders of our life and our reputations.

I believe the ideas here could literally change the world if we all applied even a part of them because the deepest longing of the human heart is to be seen, known, and, heard. Let's change the world together.

Cheering you on,

Lauren

REFERENCES

1. Keller, Timothy, and John Inazu. Uncommon Ground: Living Faithfully in a World of Difference. Thomas Nelson, 2020, p. 67.
2. Lamia, Mary C. "Emotional Memories: When People and Events Remain with You." Psychology Today, Sussex Publishers, 6 Mar. 2012, www.psychologytoday.com/us/blog/intense-emotions-and-strong-feelings/201203/emotional-memories-when-people-and-events-remain.
3. Rogers, Fred. The World According to Mister Rogers: Important Things to Remember. Hyperion, 2003.
4. Cloud, Henry. Integrity: The Courage to Face the Demands of Reality. Collins, 2006.
5. Strahan, C. R. The Roan Maverick. BookSurge, LLC, 2006.
6. Cloud, Henry. Necessary Endings: The Employees, Businesses, and Relationships That All of Us Have to Give Up in Order to Move Forward. HarperCollins, 2011.
7. Lyons, Rebekah. Rhythms of Renewal: Trading Stress and Anxiety for a Life of Peace and Purpose. Zondervan, 2019.
8. Russell, Joyce E. A. Career Coach: The Power of Using a Name - The Washington Post, 12 Jan. 2014, www.washingtonpost.com/business/capitalbusiness/career-coach-the-power-of-using-a-name/2014/01/10/8ca03da0-787e-11e3-8963-b4b654bcc9b2_story.html.

ABOUT THE AUTHOR

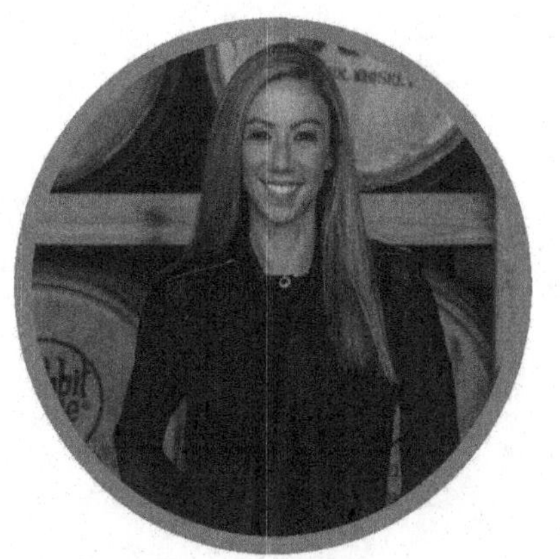

Lauren Shippy is an entrepreneur with a passion for identifying the underlying dynamics of people, products and experiences to create new ways of doing things. She has worked for multiple start ups over the years, assuming the role of COO early in her career. Lauren co-founded a family investment office with her dad out of Philadelphia, DeSimone Group Investments. Lauren now practices doing what she loves every day - providing strategy to companies of all sizes through StoryWork, her own consulting agency. She's the co-founder of The Marketing Engine + Storehouse. Additionally, Lauren loves to share her thought leadership through The Strategy Game Podcast.

She lives in Palm Beach Gardens, Florida with her husband and 2 girls.

Printed in the United States
by Baker & Taylor Publisher Services